The Ultimate Collection of Dash Diet Slow Cooker Meals

Every Day is a New Day with this Innovative Cookbook

Carmela Rojas

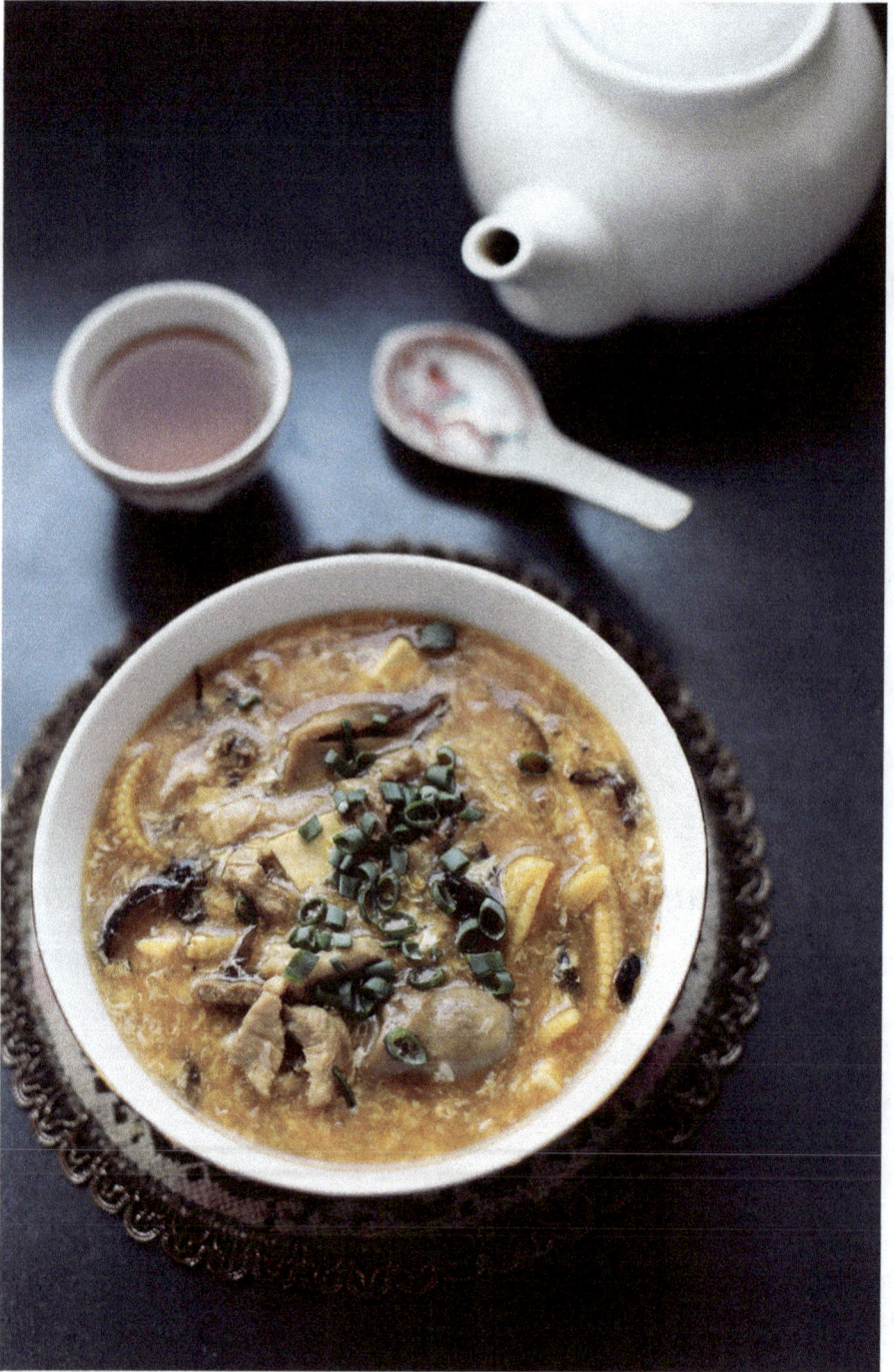

TABLE OF CONTENTS

4

Hot And Sour Soup

Servings: 4 Servings

Ingredients:

- 4 cups (950 ml) low-sodium chicken broth
- 8 ounces (225 g) bamboo shoots, drained
- ¼ cup (30 g) julienned carrot
- 8 ounces (225 g) water chestnuts, drained
- 4 ounces (115 g) mushroom, sliced
- 1 tablespoon (15 ml) rice wine vinegar
- 1 tablespoon (15 ml) low-sodium soy sauce
- ¼ teaspoon white pepper
- ¼ teaspoon red pepper flakes
- 8 ounces (225 g) shrimp, peeled
- 4 ounces (115 g) tofu, drained and cubed
- ¼ cup (60 ml) egg substitute

Directions:

1. Combine all ingredients except shrimp, tofu, and egg substitute in slow cooker. Cover and cook on low 8 to 10 hours or on high 4 to 5 hours. Add shrimp and tofu. Cover and cook 45 to 60 minutes longer. Drizzle egg substitute into the soup in a thin stream, stirring so it forms shreds.

Nutrition Info:

Per serving: 443 g water; 222 calories (17% from fat, 51% from protein, 32% from carb); 28 g protein; 4 g total fat; 1 g saturated fat; 1 g monounsaturated fat; 2 g polyunsaturated fat; 18 g carb; 2 g fiber; 4 g sugar; 360 mg phosphorus; 76 mg calcium; 3 mg iron; 320 mg sodium; 884 mg potassium; 1600 IU vitamin A; 46 mg ATE vitamin E; 5 mg vitamin C; 132 mg cholesterol

Shrimp Creole

Servings: 6 Servings

Ingredients:

- 1½ cups (150 g) sliced celery
- 1¼ cup (200 g) chopped onion
- 1 cup (150 g) chopped green bell pepper
- 1 can (8 ounces, or 225 g) no-salt-added tomato sauce
- 1 can (28 ounces, or 785 g) no-salt-added whole tomatoes, broken up
- ½ teaspoons minced garlic
- ¼ teaspoon pepper
- 6 drops hot pepper sauce
- 1 pound (455 g) shrimp, peeled

Directions:

1. Combine all ingredients except shrimp. Cook 3 to 4 hours on high or 6 to 8 hours on low. Add shrimp during the last hour of cooking. Serve over hot rice.

Nutrition Info:

Per serving: 293 g water; 139 calories (11% from fat, 50% from protein, 39% from carb); 18 g protein; 2 g total fat; 0 g saturated fat; 0 g monounsaturated fat; 1 g polyunsaturated fat; 14 g carb; 3 g fiber; 7 g sugar; 213 mg phosphorus; 106 mg calcium; 4 mg iron; 156 mg sodium; 688 mg potassium; 632 IU vitamin A; 41 mg ATE vitamin E; 42 mg vitamin C; 115 mg cholesterol

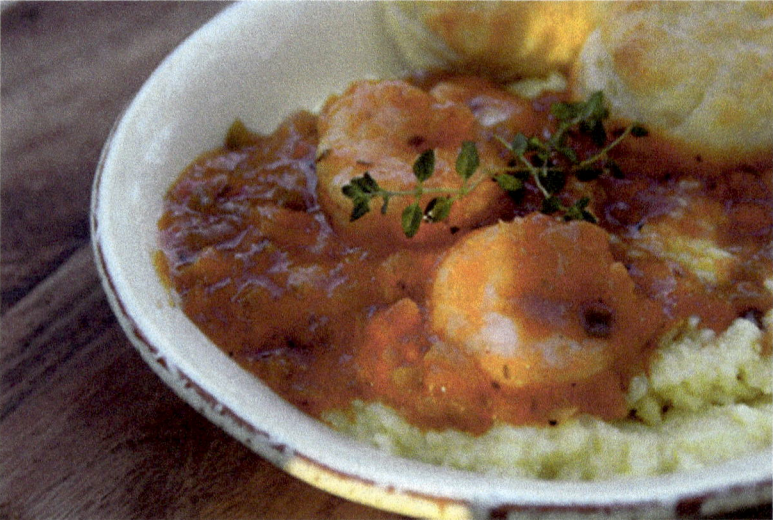

Tuna Chowder

Servings: 6 Servings

Ingredients:

- 14 ounces (390 ml) low-sodium chicken broth
- 2 medium red potatoes, chopped
- 1 can (14 ounces, or 400 g) no-salt-added diced tomatoes
- 1 cup (100 g) chopped celery
- 1 cup (160 g) chopped onion
- 1 cup (130 g) coarsely shredded carrot
- 1 teaspoon dried thyme, crushed
- 1 teaspoon cayenne pepper
- 1 teaspoon ground black pepper
- 12 ounces (340 g) water-packed tuna, drained and broken into chunks

Directions:

1. In a slow cooker, combine broth, potatoes, undrained tomatoes, celery, onion, carrot, thyme, cayenne pepper, and black pepper. Cover and cook on low for 6 to 7 hours or on high for 3 to 4 hours. Gently stir in tuna. Let stand, covered, for 5 minutes.

Nutrition Info:

Per serving: 237 g water; 149 calories (12% from fat, 42% from protein, 46% from carb); 16 g protein; 2 g total fat; 1 g saturated fat; 0 g monounsaturated fat; 1 g polyunsaturated fat; 17 g carb; 4 g fiber; 4 g sugar; 183 mg phosphorus; 63 mg calcium; 3 mg iron; 109 mg sodium; 552 mg potassium; 3883 IU vitamin A; 3 mg ATE vitamin E; 13 mg vitamin C; 24 mg cholesterol

Salmon Risotto

Servings: 4 Servings

Ingredients:

- 2 tablespoons (28 g) unsalted butter
- ¼ cup (40 g) finely chopped onion
- 8 ounces (225 g) Arborio rice
- 3 cups (705 ml) vegetable broth
- ½ cup (120 ml) dry white wine
- ¼ teaspoon freshly ground black pepper
- 1 pound (455 g) salmon fillet, cut in 1-inch (2.5 cm) cubes

Directions:

1. In a small skillet over medium-high heat, melt butter and sauté onion until softened. Transfer to slow cooker. Add remaining ingredients except salmon. Cover and cook on low 3 to 4 hours, stirring once. Stir in salmon, turn to high, and cook until fish is done and rice is tender, about 30 to 60 minutes.

Nutrition Info:

Per serving: 331 g water; 441 calories (49% from fat, 25% from protein, 26% from carb); 26 g protein; 23 g total fat; 7 g saturated fat; 8 g monounsaturated fat; 6 g polyunsaturated fat; 27 g carb; 1 g fiber; 1 g sugar; 340 mg phosphorus; 50 mg calcium; 1 mg iron; 175 mg sodium; 541 mg potassium; 237 IU vitamin A; 65 mg ATE vitamin E; 8 mg vitamin C; 82 mg cholesterol

Curried Fish

Servings: 4 Servings

Ingredients:

- 1 cup (160 g) chopped onion
- 1 tablespoon (9 g) chopped green chilies
- 1 teaspoon garlic
- 2 tablespoons (9 g) coconut
- 2/3 cup (160 ml) water, divided
- 2 tablespoons (28 ml) olive oil
- 1 tablespoon (6.3 g) mild curry powder
- 2/3 cup (160 ml) fat-free evaporated milk
- 1 pound (455 g) catfish, or other firm white fish
- 2 tablespoons (28 ml) lime juice
- 3 tablespoons (6 g) cilantro, dried

Directions:

1. Combine the onion, chilies, garlic, coconut and 3 tablespoons (45 ml) of the water. Process in a food processor until it forms a paste. Heat the oil in a skillet. Stir-fry the curry powder in the oil for a few seconds and then add the onion mixture and fry for about 5 minutes more. Stir in the remaining water

and bring to a boil. Transfer to the slow cooker and stir in the milk. Cover and cook on high for 1 hour. While the curry cooks, cut the fish into bite-size pieces. Combine the line juice and cilantro and pour over the fish to marinate for 15 minutes. Stir the fish into the sauce in the slow cooker, cover, and cook until fish flakes easily, 30 to 60 minutes.

Nutrition Info:

Per serving: 206 g water; 282 calories (53% from fat, 31% from protein, 16% from carb); 22 g protein; 16 g total fat; 4 g saturated fat; 9 g monounsaturated fat; 3 g polyunsaturated fat; 12 g carb; 1 g fiber; 7 g sugar; 335 mg phosphorus; 157 mg calcium; 1 mg iron; 123 mg sodium; 597 mg potassium; 380 IU vitamin A; 67 mg ATE vitamin E; 8 mg vitamin C; 55 mg cholesterol

Tuna Lasagna

Servings: 6 Servings

Ingredients:

- 5 tablespoons (70 g) unsalted butter, divided
- 1 cup (160 g) chopped onion
- ½ teaspoon minced garlic
- 4 ounces (115 g) mushrooms, sliced
- 1/3 cup (42 g) flour
- ¼ cup (60 ml) dry white wine
- 3 cups (705 ml) skim milk
- 1 tablespoon (1.3 g) dried parsley
- 14 ounces (390 g) tuna, in water
- 6 ounces (170 g) mozzarella, shredded
- 9 to 12 no boil lasagna noodles
- 3 tablespoons (15 g) grated Parmesan

Directions:

1. Spray the slow cooker with nonstick cooking spray. Melt 2 tablespoons (28 g) of the butter in a skillet. Sauté the onions until soft. Add the garlic and mushrooms and sauté 3 minutes more. Remove from pan. Melt the remaining butter in the skillet and stir

in the flour. Gradually stir in the wine and milk and cook until thickened. Reserve 1½ cups (355 ml) of the sauce. Add the mushroom mixture to the remaining sauce. Drain the tuna and flake and then mix the mozzarella into the tuna. Spoon a layer of the mushroom sauce in the bottom of the cooker. Cover with 3 to 4 of the noodles, breaking if necessary to fit. Cover with half of the tuna mixture, then half of the remaining mushroom sauce. Add another layer of the noodles and then repeat the tuna, mushroom sauce, and noodle layers. Pour the reserved sauce over the top and then sprinkle with the Parmesan cheese. Cover and cook on low for 2 to 3 hours or until noodles are tender.

Nutrition Info:

Per serving: 228 g water; 512 calories (33% from fat, 29% from protein, 39% from carb); 36 g protein; 18 g total fat; 10 g saturated fat; 5 g monounsaturated fat; 2 g polyunsaturated fat; 48 g carb; 2 g fiber; 2 g sugar; 472 mg phosphorus; 462 mg calcium; 3 mg iron; 336 mg sodium; 598 mg potassium; 761 IU vitamin A; 197 mg ATE vitamin E; 5 mg vitamin C; 77 mg cholesterol

Salmon Chowder

Servings: 6 Servings

Ingredients:

- 2 pounds (900 g) salmon fillets
- 1 cup (160 g) chopped onion
- 4 medium potatoes, peeled and cubed
- 2 cups (475 ml) water
- ¼ teaspoon pepper
- 12 ounces (355 ml) fat-free evaporated milk

Directions:

1. Cut salmon into bite-size pieces. Place in slow cooker. Add onion, potatoes, water, and pepper. Cover and cook on low for 5 to 8 hours. Add evaporated milk and continue cooking until heated through.

Nutrition Info:

Per serving: 451 g water; 504 calories (30% from fat, 31% from protein, 38% from carb); 39 g protein; 17 g total fat; 3 g saturated fat; 6 g monounsaturated fat; 6 g polyunsaturated fat; 48 g carb; 5 g fiber; 10 g sugar; 621 mg phosphorus; 216 mg

calcium; 3 mg iron; 173 mg sodium; 1895 mg potassium; 321 IU vitamin A; 90 mg ATE vitamin E; 30 mg vitamin C; 91 mg cholesterol

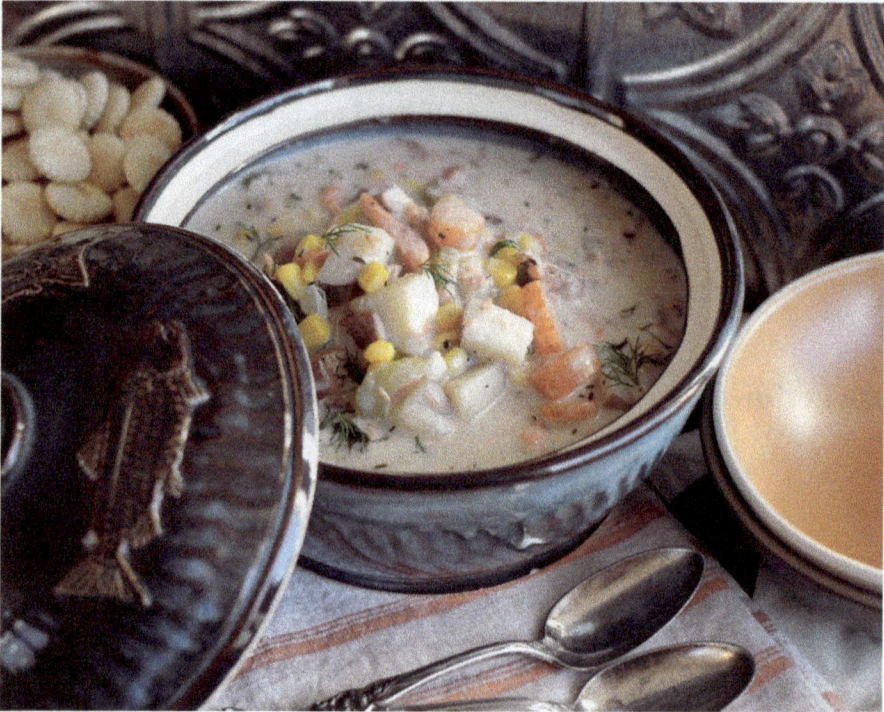

Poached Fish

Servings: 4 Servings

Ingredients:

- 1 tablespoon (15 ml) olive oil
- 1 cup (160 g) finely chopped onion
- ½ cup (120 ml) fish stock
- 1 can (8 ounces, or 225 g) no-salt-added tomato sauce
- ½ teaspoon minced garlic
- 1/8 teaspoon cumin
- 2 tablespoons (28 ml) lemon juice
- 1½ pounds (680 g) haddock, or other firm white fish

Directions:

1. Heat oil in a skillet and cook onion until soft. Bring fish stock to boiling. Combine onion, fish stock, and remaining ingredients except fish in slow cooker and cook on high until it begins to simmer around the edge, about 1½ to 2 hours. Add fish to sauce and cook until fish is tender, about 1 to 1½ hours.

Nutrition Info:

Per serving: 259 g water; 222 calories (21% from fat, 63% from protein, 16% from carb); 34 g protein; 5 g total fat; 1 g saturated fat; 3 g monounsaturated fat; 1 g polyunsaturated fat; 9 g carb; 2 g fiber; 4 g sugar; 360 mg phosphorus; 84 mg calcium; 2 mg iron; 141 mg sodium; 836 mg potassium; 298 IU vitamin A; 29 mg ATE vitamin E; 14 mg vitamin C; 97 mg cholesterol

Meatball Nibblers

Servings: 6 Servings

Ingredients:

- 2 pounds (900 g) meatballs, basic or turkey
- 1 cup (240 g) low-sodium ketchup
- 1 cup (225 g) packed brown sugar
- 1 can (6 ounces, or 170 g) no-salt-added tomato paste
- ¼ cup (60 ml) reduced-sodium soy sauce
- ¼ cup (60 ml) cider vinegar
- ½ teaspoon hot pepper sauce

Directions:

1. Preheat oven to 350°F (180°C, or gas mark 4). Place frozen meatballs on baking sheet. Bake for 18 minutes or until brown. Place meatballs in slow cooker. Combine remaining ingredients and pour over meatballs. Cover and cook on low 4 hours.

Nutrition Info:

Per serving: 157 g water; 533 calories (34% from fat, 21% from protein, 45% from carb); 28 g protein; 20 g total fat; 8 g saturated fat; 9 g monounsaturated fat; 1 g polyunsaturated fat; 61 g carb; 2 g fiber; 50 g sugar; 272 mg phosphorus; 112 mg calcium; 5 mg iron; 194 mg sodium; 1023 mg potassium; 898 IU vitamin A; 14 mg ATE vitamin E; 12 mg vitamin C; 80 mg cholesterol

Cranberry Orange Meatballs

Servings: 4 Servings

Ingredients:

- 2 tablespoons (28 ml) olive oil
- 1 cup (160 g) finely chopped onion
- 1 pound (455 g) jellied cranberry sauce
- 1 pound (455 g) meatballs, basic or turkey
- 1 teaspoon orange peel

Directions:

1. In small saucepan, heat oil over medium-high heat and sauté onion. Stir cranberry sauce into saucepan. Heat on low until melted. Combine cranberry mixture and remaining ingredients in slow cooker. Cover and cook on low 2 to 4 hours.

Nutrition Info:

Per serving: 173 g water; 491 calories (40% from fat, 16% from protein, 44% from carb); 20 g protein; 22 g total fat; 7 g saturated fat; 12 g monounsaturated fat; 2 g polyunsaturated fat; 55 g carb; 3 g fiber; 46 g sugar; 180 mg phosphorus; 60 mg calcium; 3 mg iron; 116 mg sodium; 411 mg potassium; 115 IU vitamin A; 11 mg ATE vitamin E; 6 mg vitamin C; 60 mg cholesterol

Sour Cream Meatballs

Servings: 6 Servings

Ingredients:

- 2 pounds (900 g) meatballs, basic or turkey
- ¼ cup (31 g) flour
- ¼ teaspoon garlic powder
- ¼ teaspoon pepper
- 1 teaspoon paprika
- 2 cups (475 ml) boiling water
- ¾ cup (180 g) fat-free sour cream

Directions:

1. Brown meatballs in skillet. Reserve drippings and place meatballs in slow cooker. Cover and cook on high 10 to 15 minutes. Stir flour, garlic powder, pepper, and paprika into hot drippings in skillet. Stir in water and sour cream. Pour sour cream mixture over meatballs in slow cooker. Cover, reduce heat to low, and cook 4 to 5 hours.

Nutrition Info:

Per serving: 195 g water; 386 calories (57% from fat, 28% from protein, 15% from carb); 27 g protein; 24 g total fat; 10 g saturated fat; 10 g monounsaturated fat; 1 g polyunsaturated fat; 15 g carb; 1 g fiber; 2 g sugar; 251 mg phosphorus; 96 mg calcium; 3 mg iron; 123 mg sodium; 485 mg potassium; 404 IU vitamin A; 44 mg ATE vitamin E; 1 mg vitamin C; 91 mg cholesterol

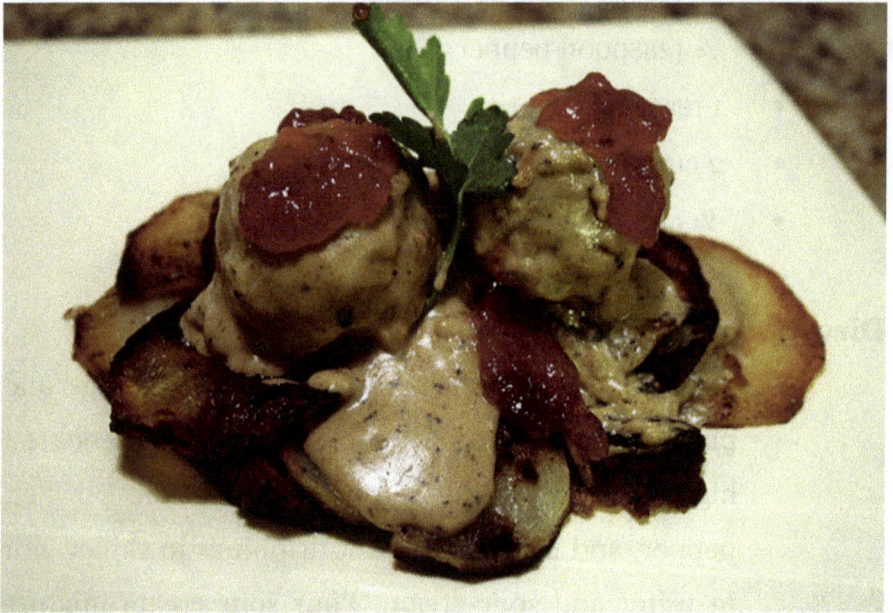

Stuffed Peppers

Servings: 6 Servings

Ingredients:

- 6 green bell peppers
- 1 pound (455 g) extra-lean ground beef
- ½ cup (80 g) chopped onions
- ¼ teaspoon black pepper
- 1½ cups (250 g) cooked rice
- 2 tablespoons (28 ml) Worcestershire sauce
- 1 cup (245 g) no-salt-added tomato sauce

Directions:

1. Cut tops from peppers. Carefully remove seeds and membrane. Brown ground beef and onions in skillet over medium-high heat. Drain. Place meat and onions in mixing bowl. Add pepper, rice, and Worcestershire sauce to meat and combine well. Stuff green peppers with mixture. Stand stuffed peppers upright in slow cooker. Pour tomato sauce over peppers. Cover and cook on low 5 to 7 hours.

Nutrition Info:

Per serving: 262 g water; 282 calories (43% from fat, 24% from protein, 33% from carb); 17 g protein; 13 g total fat; 5 g saturated fat; 6 g monounsaturated fat; 1 g polyunsaturated fat; 23 g carb; 4 g fiber; 6 g sugar; 175 mg phosphorus; 33 mg calcium; 3 mg iron; 108 mg sodium; 690 mg potassium; 688 IU vitamin A; 0 mg ATE vitamin E; 135 mg vitamin C; 52 mg cholesterol

Turkey Meat Loaf

Servings: 8 Servings

Ingredients:

- 1½ pounds (680 g) ground turkey
- 1 cup (160 g) chopped onion
- ½ cup (120 ml) egg substitute
- 2/3 cup (53 g) quick-cooking oats
- 2 tablespoons (15 g) onion soup mix
- ¼ teaspoon liquid smoke
- 1 teaspoon dry mustard
- 1 cup (240 g) low-sodium ketchup, divided

Directions:

1. Mix turkey and chopped onion thoroughly. Combine with egg substitute, oats, dry soup mix, liquid smoke, mustard, and all but 2 tablespoons (30 g) of ketchup. Shape into loaf and place in slow cooker sprayed with nonstick cooking spray. Top meat loaf with remaining ketchup. Cover and cook on low 8 to 10 hours or on high 4 to 6 hours.

Nutrition Info:

Per serving: 107 g water; 221 calories (22% from fat, 52% from protein, 26% from carb); 29 g protein; 5 g total fat; 2 g saturated fat; 1 g monounsaturated fat; 2 g polyunsaturated fat; 14 g carb; 1 g fiber; 8 g sugar; 248 mg phosphorus; 43 mg calcium; 2 mg iron; 94 mg sodium; 474 mg potassium; 337 IU vitamin A; 0 mg ATE vitamin E; 6 mg vitamin C; 65 mg cholesterol

Meat Loaf

Servings: 8 Servings

Ingredients:

- 2 pounds (900 g) extra-lean ground beef
- ½ cup (120 ml) egg substitute
- 2/3 cup (53 g) quick-cooking or rolled oats
- 2 tablespoons (15 g) low-sodium onion soup mix
- ½ cup (120 g) low-sodium ketchup, divided

Directions:

1. Combine ground beef, egg substitute, oats, soup mix, and all but 2 tablespoons (30 g) ketchup. Shape into loaf and place in slow cooker. Top with remaining 2 tablespoons (30 g) ketchup. Cover and cook on low for 6 to 8 hours or on high for 2 to 4 hours.

Nutrition Info:

Per serving: 96 g water; 318 calories (58% from fat, 31% from protein, 11% from carb); 24 g protein; 20 g total fat; 8 g saturated fat; 9 g monounsaturated fat; 1 g polyunsaturated fat; 8 g carb; 1 g fiber; 4 g sugar; 214 mg phosphorus; 22 mg

calcium; 3 mg iron; 106 mg sodium; 455 mg potassium; 196 IU vitamin A; 0 mg ATE vitamin E; 2 mg vitamin C; 78 mg cholesterol

Cornbread Casserole

Servings: 6 Servings

Ingredients:

- 1 pound (455 g) frozen corn
- 1 cup (140 g) cornmeal
- ½ teaspoon baking soda
- ¼ cup (60 ml) canola oil
- 1 cup (235 ml) skim milk
- ½ cup (120 ml) egg substitute
- ¼ cup (65 g) low-sodium salsa
- 1 cup (115 g) shredded Cheddar cheese
- 1 cup (160 g) chopped onion
- ½ teaspoon minced garlic
- 4 ounces (115 g) diced green chilies
- 1 pound (455 g) extra-lean ground beef, lightly cooked and drained

Directions:

1. Combine corn, cornmeal, baking soda, oil, milk, egg substitute, and salsa. Pour half of mixture into slow cooker. Layer cheese, onion, garlic, green chilies, and ground beef on top of cornmeal mixture. Cover with

remaining cornmeal mixture. Cover and cook on high 1 hour and then on low for 3 to 4 hours or only on low for 6 hours.

Nutrition Info:

Per serving: 222 g water; 559 calories (50% from fat, 20% from protein, 30% from carb); 28 g protein; 31 g total fat; 11 g saturated fat; 14 g monounsaturated fat; 4 g polyunsaturated fat; 43 g carb; 4 g fiber; 5 g sugar; 375 mg phosphorus; 254 mg calcium; 4 mg iron; 354 mg sodium; 625 mg potassium; 494 IU vitamin A; 82 mg ATE vitamin E; 12 mg vitamin C; 76 mg cholesterol

Cowboy Meal

Servings: 5 Servings

Ingredients:

- 1 pound (455 g) extra-lean ground beef, browned
- 15 ounces (425 g) frozen corn
- 2 cups (512 g) no-salt-added kidney beans
- 1 can (10 ounces, or 280 g) reduced-sodium condensed tomato soup
- 1 cup (115 g) shredded Cheddar cheese
- ¼ cup (60 ml) milk
- 1 teaspoon onion flakes
- ½ teaspoon chili powder

Directions:

1. Combine all ingredients in slow cooker. Cover and cook on low for 1 hour.

Nutrition Info:

Per serving: 241 g water; 506 calories (45% from fat, 26% from protein, 29% from carb); 34 g protein; 26 g total fat; 12 g saturated fat; 10 g monounsaturated fat; 2 g polyunsaturated fat; 37 g carb; 9 g fiber; 5 g sugar; 458 mg phosphorus; 265 mg

calcium; 5 mg iron; 258 mg sodium; 900 mg potassium; 692 IU vitamin A; 79 mg ATE vitamin E; 22 mg vitamin C; 91 mg cholesterol

Creamy Ground Beef And Vegetables

Servings: 8 Servings

Ingredients:

- 1 pound (455 g) ground beef
- 1 cup (160 g) sliced onions
- 1 cup (130 g) thinly sliced carrots
- 1/8 teaspoon pepper
- 10 ounces (280 g) low-sodium cream of mushroom soup
- ¼ cup (60 ml) milk
- 4 potatoes, thinly sliced

Directions:

1. Spray slow cooker with nonstick cooking spray. Layer ground beef, onions, carrots, and pepper in prepared slow cooker. Combine soup and milk. Toss with potatoes. Arrange potato mixture in slow cooker. Cover and cook on low 7 to 9 hours.

Nutrition Info:

Per serving: 255 g water; 297 calories (32% from fat, 20% from protein, 48% from carb); 15 g protein; 11 g total fat; 4 g saturated fat; 4 g monounsaturated fat; 1 g polyunsaturated fat; 36 g carb; 4 g fiber; 5 g sugar; 230 mg phosphorus; 46 mg calcium; 3 mg iron; 199 mg sodium; 1225 mg potassium; 2723 IU vitamin A; 5 mg ATE vitamin E; 18 mg vitamin C; 40 mg cholesterol

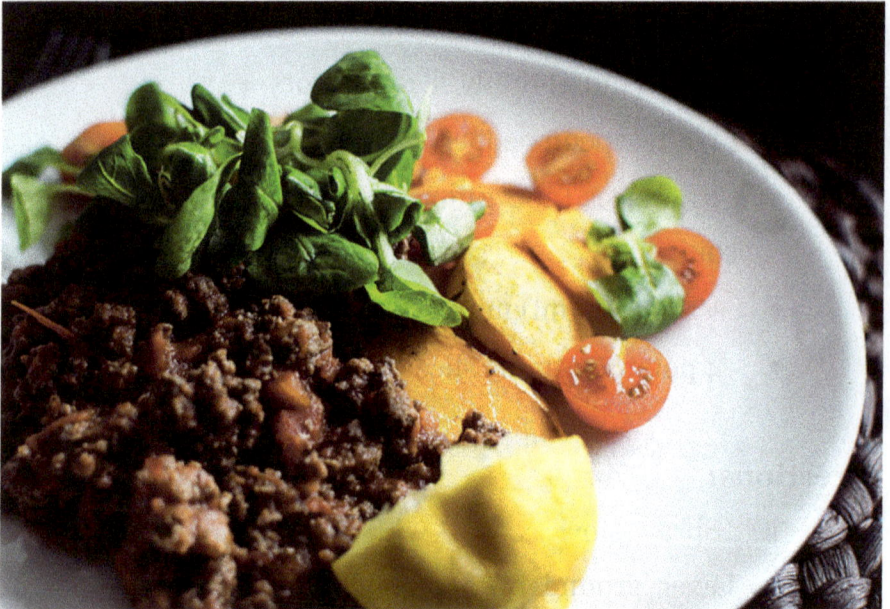

Barbecued Beef

Servings: 12 Servings

Ingredients:

- 3 pounds (1 1/3 kg) extra-lean ground beef
- 1 cup (250 g) barbecue sauce
- ½ cup (160 g) apricot preserves
- ½ cup (75 g) finely chopped green bell pepper
- ½ cup (80 g) finely chopped onion
- 1 tablespoon (11 g) Dijon mustard
- 1 tablespoon (15 g) brown sugar

Directions:

1. Spray slow cooker with nonstick cooking spray. Place meat in prepared slow cooker. Combine barbecue sauce, preserves, green pepper, onion, mustard, and brown sugar. Pour over meat. Cover and cook on low 6 to 8 hours.

Nutrition Info:

Per serving: 101 g water; 353 calories (50% from fat, 25% from protein, 25% from carb); 22 g protein; 19 g total fat; 8 g saturated fat; 8 g monounsaturated fat; 1 g polyunsaturated fat;

21 g carb; 0 g fiber; 16 g sugar; 167 mg phosphorus; 14 mg calcium; 2 mg iron; 114 mg sodium; 359 mg potassium; 24 IU vitamin A; 0 mg ATE vitamin E; 7 mg vitamin C; 78 mg cholesterol

Hamburger Stew

Servings: 8 Servings

Ingredients:

- 2 pounds (900 g) extra-lean ground beef
- 1 cup (160 g) chopped onion
- ½ teaspoon minced garlic
- 2 cups (475 ml) low-sodium tomato juice
- 1 cup (130 g) sliced carrots
- ½ cup (50 g) sliced celery
- ½ cup (75 g) chopped green bell pepper
- 2 cups (248 g) frozen green beans
- 2 medium potatoes, cubed
- 2 cups (475 ml) water
- 1 tablespoon (15 ml) Worcestershire sauce
- ¼ teaspoon oregano
- ½ teaspoon basil
- ¼ teaspoon thyme
- 1 tablespoon (7 g) low-sodium onion soup mix
- ¼ teaspoon pepper

Directions:

1. Brown meat and onion in saucepan over medium-high heat. Drain. Stir in garlic and tomato juice. Heat to boiling. Combine meat mixture and remaining ingredients in slow cooker. Cover and cook on low 8 to 10 hours.

Nutrition Info:

Per serving: 335 g water; 368 calories (48% from fat, 26% from protein, 26% from carb); 24 g protein; 20 g total fat; 8 g saturated fat; 8 g monounsaturated fat; 1 g polyunsaturated fat; 24 g carb; 4 g fiber; 5 g sugar; 255 mg phosphorus; 51 mg calcium; 4 mg iron; 126 mg sodium; 1070 mg potassium; 3235 IU vitamin A; 0 mg ATE vitamin E; 37 mg vitamin C; 78 mg cholesterol

Sweet And Sour Meatballs

Servings: 6 Servings

Ingredients:

- 2 pounds (900 g) meatballs, basic or turkey
- 1 cup (165 g) pineapple chunks, juice reserved
- 3 tablespoons (24 g) cornstarch
- ¼ cup (60 ml) cold water
- 1 cup (240 g) low-sodium ketchup
- ¼ cup (60 ml) Worcestershire sauce
- ¼ teaspoon pepper
- ¼ teaspoon garlic powder
- ½ cup (75 g) chopped green bell pepper

Directions:

1. Brown meatballs in a skillet over medium-high heat, rolling so all sides are browned. Place meatballs in slow cooker. Pour juice from pineapple chunks into skillet. Stir into drippings. Combine cornstarch and cold water. Add to skillet and stir until thickened. Stir in ketchup and Worcestershire sauce and then add pepper and garlic powder. Add green pepper and pineapple chunks. Pour pineapple mixture over meatballs. Cover and cook on low 6 hours.

Nutrition Info:

Per serving: 180 g water; 403 calories (45% from fat, 26% from protein, 28% from carb); 26 g protein; 20 g total fat; 8 g saturated fat; 9 g monounsaturated fat; 1 g polyunsaturated fat; 29 g carb; 2 g fiber; 15 g sugar; 244 mg phosphorus; 76 mg calcium; 4 mg iron; 215 mg sodium; 738 mg potassium; 535 IU vitamin A; 14 mg ATE vitamin E; 37 mg vitamin C; 80 mg cholesterol

Barbecue Burgers

Servings: 8 Servings

Ingredients:

- 2 tablespoons (28 ml) olive oil
- 1½ pounds (680 g) extra-lean ground beef
- ½ cup (80 g) chopped onions
- ½ cup (50 g) diced celery
- ½ cup (75 g) chopped green bell pepper
- 1 tablespoon (15 ml) Worcestershire sauce
- ½ cup (120 g) low-sodium ketchup
- ½ teaspoon minced garlic
- ¼ teaspoon pepper
- ½ teaspoon paprika
- 1 can (6 ounces, or 170 g) no-salt-added tomato paste
- 2 tablespoons (28 ml) vinegar
- 2 teaspoons brown sugar
- 1 teaspoon dry mustard

Directions:

1. Heat oil in a saucepan over medium-high heat and brown beef. Drain. Combine beef and remaining

ingredients in slow cooker. Cover and cook on low 6 to 8 hours or on high 3 to 4 hours.

Nutrition Info:

Per serving: 108 g water; 276 calories (59% from fat, 25% from protein, 16% from carb); 17 g protein; 18 g total fat; 6 g saturated fat; 9 g monounsaturated fat; 1 g polyunsaturated fat; 11 g carb; 1 g fiber; 8 g sugar; 152 mg phosphorus; 24 mg calcium; 3 mg iron; 105 mg sodium; 589 mg potassium; 609 IU vitamin A; 0 mg ATE vitamin E; 19 mg vitamin C; 59 mg cholesterol

Taco Filling

Servings: 8 Servings

Ingredients:

- 3 tablespoons (45 ml) olive oil
- 2 pounds (900 g) extra-lean ground beef
- 1 cup (160 g) chopped onion
- 8 ounces (225 g) diced green chilies
- 1 teaspoon chili powder
- 1 teaspoon minced garlic
- 1 cup (235 ml) water

Directions:

1. Heat oil in a large skillet over medium-high heat; brown meat and onion. Transfer to slow cooker. Add chilies, chili powder, garlic, and water. Cover and cook on high 6 to 8 hours.

Nutrition Info:

Per serving: 146 g water; 326 calories (69% from fat, 27% from protein, 4% from carb); 22 g protein; 25 g total fat; 8 g saturated fat; 12 g monounsaturated fat; 1 g polyunsaturated fat; 3 g carb; 1 g fiber; 1 g sugar; 170 mg phosphorus; 25 mg calcium; 3 mg

iron; 192 mg sodium; 391 mg potassium; 129 IU vitamin A; 0 mg ATE vitamin E; 11 mg vitamin C; 78 mg cholesterol

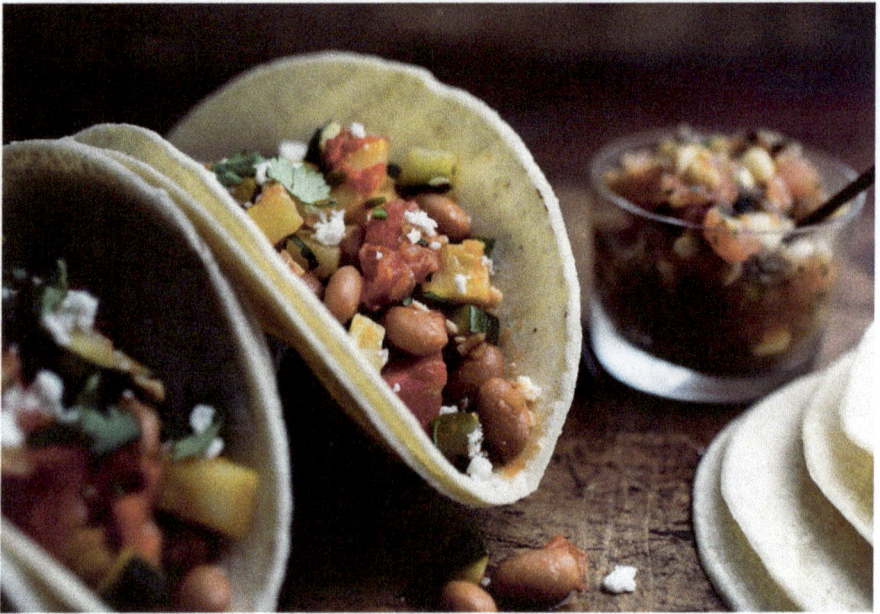

Stuffed Peppers With Beef And Corn

Servings: 6 Servings

Ingredients:

- 6 green bell peppers
- 1 pound (455 g) extra-lean ground beef, browned
- ½ cup (80 g) chopped onion
- ¼ teaspoon black pepper
- 12 ounces (340 g) frozen corn
- 1 tablespoon (15 ml) Worcestershire sauce
- 1 teaspoon mustard
- 1 can (10 ounces, or 280 g) reduced-sodium condensed tomato soup

Directions:

1. Cut off the top of each pepper. Remove core, seeds, and white membrane from each. In a small bowl, combine beef, onions, pepper, and corn. Divide evenly among peppers. Stand peppers up in slow cooker. Combine Worcestershire sauce, mustard, and

tomato soup. Pour over peppers. Cover and cook on low 5 to 6 hours.

Nutrition Info:

Per serving: 286 g water; 280 calories (44% from fat, 25% from protein, 31% from carb); 18 g protein; 14 g total fat; 5 g saturated fat; 6 g monounsaturated fat; 1 g polyunsaturated fat; 23 g carb; 4 g fiber; 7 g sugar; 200 mg phosphorus; 28 mg calcium; 3 mg iron; 97 mg sodium; 722 mg potassium; 797 IU vitamin A; 3 mg ATE vitamin E; 142 mg vitamin C; 52 mg cholesterol

Basic Turkey Meatballs

Servings: 8 Servings

Ingredients:

- 2 pounds (900 g) ground turkey
- ½ cup (120 ml) egg substitute
- ¾ cup (90 g) bread crumbs
- ½ cup (80 g) finely chopped onion
- 1 teaspoon parsley
- ¼ teaspoon black pepper
- ¼ teaspoon garlic powder

Directions:

1. Combine all ingredients. Shape into walnut-sized balls. Place on waxed paper-lined cookie sheets. Freeze. When fully frozen, place in a resealable plastic bag and store in freezer until needed. When ready to use, place frozen meatballs in slow cooker. Cover and cook on high as you mix up the sauce or whatever accompaniment you are using.

Nutrition Info:

Per serving: 96 g water; 250 calories (25% from fat, 61% from protein, 14% from carb); 37 g protein; 7 g total fat; 2 g saturated fat; 1 g monounsaturated fat; 2 g polyunsaturated fat; 8 g carb; 1 g fiber; 1 g sugar; 281 mg phosphorus; 58 mg calcium; 3 mg iron; 108 mg sodium; 427 mg potassium; 70 IU vitamin A; 0 mg ATE vitamin E; 1 mg vitamin C; 86 mg cholesterol

Basic Meatballs

Servings: 12 Servings

Ingredients:

- 3 pounds (1 1/3 kg) extra-lean ground beef
- 5 ounces (150 ml) fat-free evaporated milk
- 1 cup (80 g) rolled or quick cooking oats
- 1 cup (100 g) cracker crumbs
- ½ cup (120 ml) egg substitute
- ½ cup (80 g) chopped onion
- ½ teaspoon garlic powder
- ½ teaspoon black pepper

Directions:

1. Combine all ingredients. Shape into walnut-sized balls. Place on waxed paper-lined cookie sheets. Freeze. When fully frozen, place in a resealable plastic bag and store in freezer until needed. When ready to use, place frozen meatballs in slow cooker. Cover and cook on high as you mix up the sauce or whatever accompaniment you are using.

Nutrition Info:

Per serving: 96 g water; 322 calories (58% from fat, 31% from protein, 11% from carb); 25 g protein; 20 g total fat; 8 g saturated fat; 9 g monounsaturated fat; 1 g polyunsaturated fat; 9 g carb; 1 g fiber; 2 g sugar; 213 mg phosphorus; 66 mg calcium; 3 mg iron; 107 mg sodium; 426 mg potassium; 85 IU vitamin A; 14 mg ATE vitamin E; 1 mg vitamin C; 79 mg cholesterol

Meat Loaf Meal

Servings: 6 Servings

Ingredients:

- 6 medium potatoes, cubed
- 1 cup (130 g) thinly sliced carrots
- ¼ cup (60 ml) egg substitute
- ¼ cup (25 g) cracker crumbs
- ¼ cup (70 g) chili sauce
- ¼ cup (40 g) finely chopped onion
- ¼ teaspoon marjoram
- 1 teaspoon pepper
- 1 pound (455 g) extra-lean ground beef

Directions:

1. Place potatoes and carrots in slow cooker. Combine egg substitute, cracker crumbs, chili sauce, onion, marjoram, and pepper. Add ground beef and mix well. Shape into a loaf slightly smaller in diameter than the cooker. Place on top of vegetables, not touching sides of cooker. Cover and cook on low 9 to 10 hours.

Nutrition Info:

Per serving: 390 g water; 478 calories (26% from fat, 19% from protein, 54% from carb); 23 g protein; 14 g total fat; 5 g saturated fat; 6 g monounsaturated fat; 1 g polyunsaturated fat; 66 g carb; 7 g fiber; 6 g sugar; 361 mg phosphorus; 67 mg calcium; 5 mg iron; 114 mg sodium; 2016 mg potassium; 3835 IU vitamin A; 0 mg ATE vitamin E; 36 mg vitamin C; 52 mg cholesterol

Cranberry Salsa Meatballs

Servings: 6 Servings

Ingredients:

- 2 cups (520 g) low-sodium salsa
- 1 pound (455 g) jellied cranberry sauce
- 2 pounds (900 g) meatballs, basic or turkey

Directions:

1. Melt cranberry sauce in saucepan. Stir in salsa and meatballs. Bring to boil. Stir. Pour into slow cooker. Cover and cook on low 6 to 8 hours.

Nutrition Info:

Per serving: 205 g water; 459 calories (40% from fat, 23% from protein, 37% from carb); 27 g protein; 20 g total fat; 8 g saturated fat; 9 g monounsaturated fat; 1 g polyunsaturated fat; 43 g carb; 3 g fiber; 33 g sugar; 243 mg phosphorus; 84 mg calcium; 4 mg iron; 305 mg sodium; 674 mg potassium; 338 IU vitamin A; 14 mg ATE vitamin E; 3 mg vitamin C; 80 mg cholesterol

Hamburger Noodle Casserole

Servings: 8 Servings

Ingredients:

- 1½ pounds (680 g) extra-lean ground beef, browned and drained
- 1 cup (150 g) diced green bell pepper
- 4 cups (720 g) no-salt-added diced tomatoes
- 10 ounces (280 g) low-sodium cream of mushroom soup
- 1 cup (160 g) diced onion
- 8 ounces (225 g) uncooked egg noodles
- ¼ teaspoon black pepper
- 1 cup (110 g) shredded Swiss cheese

Directions:

1. Combine all ingredients except cheese in slow cooker. Cover and cook on high 3 to 4 hours. Sprinkle with cheese before serving.

Nutrition Info:

Per serving: 259 g water; 348 calories (52% from fat, 26% from protein, 22% from carb); 23 g protein; 20 g total fat; 9 g saturated fat; 8 g monounsaturated fat; 1 g polyunsaturated fat; 19 g carb; 3 g fiber; 5 g sugar; 292 mg phosphorus; 213 mg calcium; 3 mg iron; 211 mg sodium; 689 mg potassium; 364 IU vitamin A; 36 mg ATE vitamin E; 28 mg vitamin C; 75 mg cholesterol

Sloppy J.

Servings: 4 Servings

Ingredients:

- 1 pound (455 g) extra-lean ground beef
- 1 cup (160 g) chopped onion
- ¾ cup (180 g) low-sodium ketchup
- 2 tablespoons (40 g) chili sauce
- 1 tablespoon (15 ml) Worcestershire sauce
- 1 tablespoon (11 g) mustard
- 1 tablespoon (15 ml) vinegar

Directions:

1. Brown beef and onion in saucepan over medium-high heat. Drain. Combine beef mixture and remaining ingredients in slow cooker. Cover and cook on low 4 to 5 hours. Serve on buns.

Nutrition Info:

Per serving: 150 g water; 335 calories (53% from fat, 27% from protein, 20% from carb); 23 g protein; 20 g total fat; 8 g saturated fat; 8 g monounsaturated fat; 1 g polyunsaturated fat; 17 g carb; 1 g fiber; 12 g sugar; 191 mg phosphorus; 30 mg

calcium; 3 mg iron; 128 mg sodium; 592 mg potassium; 553 IU vitamin A; 0 mg ATE vitamin E; 18 mg vitamin C; 78 mg cholesterol

Italian Meat Loaf

Servings: 8 Servings

Ingredients:

- 2 pounds (900 g) extra-lean ground beef
- 2 cups (230 g) bread crumbs
- ½ cup (123 g) low-sodium spaghetti sauce
- ¼ cup (60 ml) egg substitute
- 1 tablespoon (15 g) onion flakes
- ¼ teaspoon pepper
- 1 teaspoon garlic powder
- 1 teaspoon Italian seasoning

Directions:

1. Fold a 30-inch (75 cm) long piece of foil in half lengthwise. Place in bottom of slow cooker with both ends hanging over the edge of cooker. Spray foil with nonstick cooking spray. Combine all ingredients and shape into a loaf. Place on top of foil in slow cooker. Cover and cook on high for 2½ to 3 hours or on low for 5 to 6 hours.

Nutrition Info:

Per serving: 92 g water; 399 calories (50% from fat, 27% from protein, 23% from carb); 26 g protein; 22 g total fat; 8 g saturated fat; 9 g monounsaturated fat; 2 g polyunsaturated fat; 23 g carb; 2 g fiber; 4 g sugar; 223 mg phosphorus; 70 mg calcium; 4 mg iron; 94 mg sodium; 477 mg potassium; 136 IU vitamin A; 0 mg ATE vitamin E; 2 mg vitamin C; 78 mg cholesterol

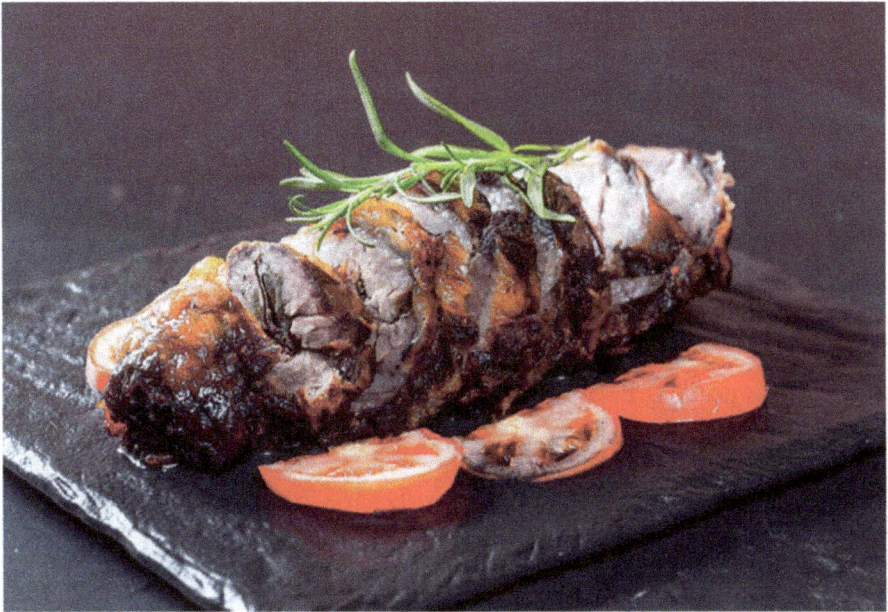

Barbecued Meatballs

Servings: 6 Servings

Ingredients:

- 2 pounds (900 g) meatballs, basic or turkey
- 1 cup (240 g) low-sodium ketchup
- ½ cup (115 g) brown sugar
- ½ teaspoon liquid smoke
- ½ teaspoon garlic powder
- ½ cup (80 g) chopped onion

Directions:

1. Place frozen meatballs in slow cooker. Cover and cook on high as you mix the remaining ingredients. Pour ketchup mixture over meatballs. Stir, cover, and continue cooking on high for 1 hour. Stir, turn to low, and cook 6 to 9 hours.

Nutrition Info:

Per serving: 131 g water; 439 calories (41% from fat, 24% from protein, 35% from carb); 26 g protein; 20 g total fat; 8 g saturated fat; 9 g monounsaturated fat; 1 g polyunsaturated fat; 38 g carb; 1 g fiber; 29 g sugar; 237 mg phosphorus; 87 mg

calcium; 4 mg iron; 124 mg sodium; 668 mg potassium; 459 IU vitamin A; 14 mg ATE vitamin E; 7 mg vitamin C; 80 mg cholesterol

Spanish Rice With Beef

Servings: 8 Servings

Ingredients:

- 2 pounds (900 g) extra-lean ground beef, browned
- 1½ cups (240 g) chopped onions
- 1½ cups (225 g) chopped green bell pepper
- 1 can (28 ounces, or 785 g) no-salt-added diced tomatoes
- 1 cup (245 g) no-salt-added tomato sauce
- 1½ cups (355 ml) water
- 2 teaspoons Worcestershire sauce
- 1½ cups (278 g) uncooked long-grain rice

Directions:

1. Combine all ingredients in slow cooker. Cover and cook on low 8 to 10 hours or on high 6 hours.

Nutrition Info:

Per serving: 410 g water; 438 calories (41% from fat, 23% from protein, 35% from carb); 25 g protein; 20 g total fat; 8 g saturated fat; 9 g monounsaturated fat; 1 g polyunsaturated fat; 38 g carb; 3 g fiber; 6 g sugar; 243 mg phosphorus; 67 mg

calcium; 5 mg iron; 112 mg sodium; 758 mg potassium; 320 IU vitamin A; 0 mg ATE vitamin E; 40 mg vitamin C; 78 mg cholesterol

Creamy Hamburger Sauce

Servings: 8 Servings

Ingredients:

- 1 pound (455 g) extra-lean ground beef
- 2 cups (220 g) shredded Swiss cheese
- 1 cup (160 g) diced onion
- 1 can (10 ounces, or 280 g) low-sodium cream of mushroom soup
- 1 can (12 ounces, or 340 g) no-salt-added diced tomatoes, undrained

Directions:

1. Brown ground beef in a nonstick skillet over medium-high heat. Drain. Combine beef and remaining ingredients in slow cooker. Cook on low 3 to 5 hours or until heated through.

Nutrition Info:

Per serving: 137 g water; 290 calories (60% from fat, 29% from protein, 10% from carb); 21 g protein; 19 g total fat; 10 g saturated fat; 7 g monounsaturated fat; 1 g polyunsaturated fat; 8 g carb; 1 g fiber; 3 g sugar; 312 mg phosphorus; 343 mg

calcium; 2 mg iron; 184 mg sodium; 439 mg potassium; 323 IU vitamin A; 70 mg ATE vitamin E; 5 mg vitamin C; 71 mg cholesterol

Goulash

Servings: 8 Servings

Ingredients:

- 1 pound (455 g) extra-lean ground beef, browned
- 1 cup (160 g) chopped onion
- ½ teaspoon minced garlic
- ½ cup (120 g) low-sodium ketchup
- 2 tablespoons (28 ml) Worcestershire sauce
- 1 tablespoon (15 g) brown sugar
- 2 teaspoons paprika
- ½ teaspoon dry mustard
- 1 cup (235 ml) water

Directions:

1. Place meat in slow cooker. Cover with onions. Combine remaining ingredients and pour over meat. Cook on low for 5 to 6 hours.

Nutrition Info:

Per serving: 95 g water; 167 calories (53% from fat, 27% from protein, 20% from carb); 11 g protein; 10 g total fat; 4 g saturated fat; 4 g monounsaturated fat; 0 g polyunsaturated fat;

8 g carb; 1 g fiber; 6 g sugar; 97 mg phosphorus; 15 mg calcium; 2 mg iron; 80 mg sodium; 299 mg potassium; 448 IU vitamin A; 0 mg ATE vitamin E; 11 mg vitamin C; 39 mg cholesterol

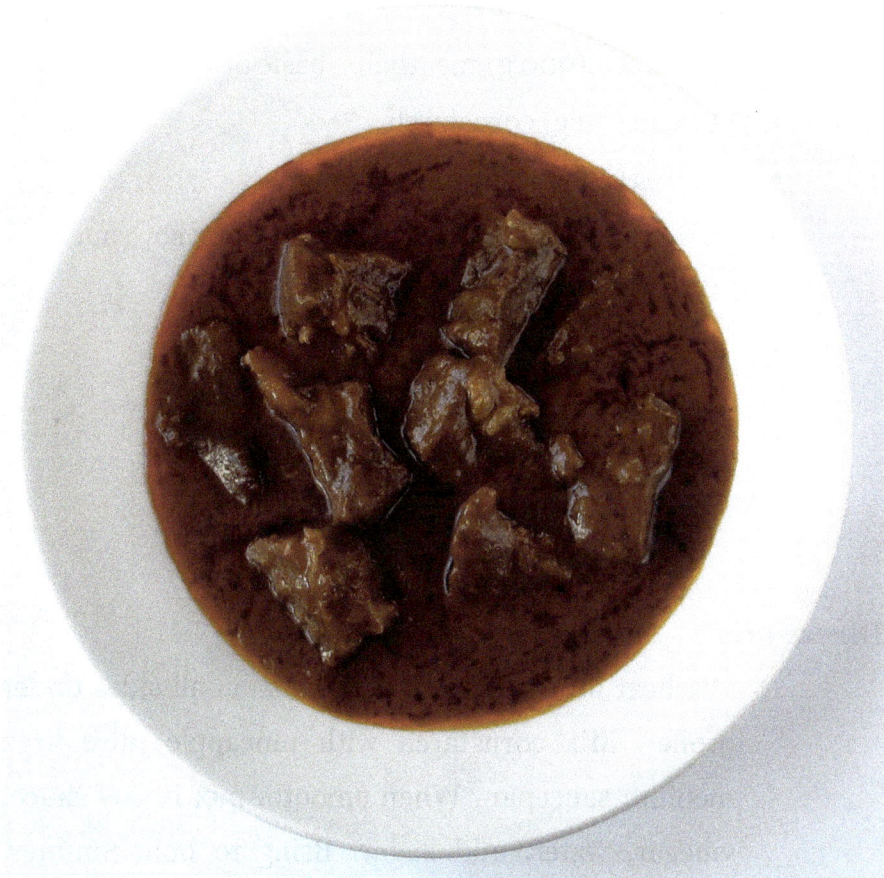

Asian Meatballs

Servings: 6 Servings

Ingredients:

- 2 pounds (900 g) meatballs, basic or turkey
- ¼ cup (30 g) cornstarch
- 2 cups (475 ml) pineapple juice
- 2 tablespoons (28 ml) reduced-sodium soy sauce
- ½ cup (120 ml) red wine vinegar
- ¾ cup (175 ml) water
- ½ cup (100 g) sugar
- 1 cup (150 g) green bell pepper strips
- 6 ounces (170 g) water chestnuts, drained

Directions:

1. Preheat broiler. Brown meatballs on all sides under broiler. Mix cornstarch with pineapple juice in a medium saucepan. When smooth, mix in soy sauce, vinegar, water, and sugar. Bring to boil. Simmer, stirring until thickened. Combine meatballs and sauce in slow cooker. Cover and cook on low 2 hours. Add green pepper and water chestnuts. Cover and cook 1 hour.

Nutrition Info:

Per serving: 259 g water; 493 calories (37% from fat, 22% from protein, 41% from carb); 26 g protein; 20 g total fat; 8 g saturated fat; 9 g monounsaturated fat; 1 g polyunsaturated fat; 50 g carb; 3 g fiber; 29 g sugar; 252 mg phosphorus; 80 mg calcium; 4 mg iron; 134 mg sodium; 765 mg potassium; 182 IU vitamin A; 14 mg ATE vitamin E; 30 mg vitamin C; 80 mg cholesterol

Enchilada Casserole

Servings: 8 Servings

Ingredients:

- 1 pound (455 g) extra-lean ground beef
- 1 cup (160 g) chopped onion
- ¾ cup (113 g) chopped green bell pepper
- 2 cups (342 g) no-salt-added cooked pinto beans
- 2 cups (344 g) no-salt-added cooked black beans
- 2 cups (360 g) no-salt-added diced tomatoes
- 4 ounces (115 g) diced green chilies
- 1 teaspoon chili powder
- 1 teaspoon ground cumin
- ½ teaspoon black pepper
- 4 ounces (115 g) Cheddar cheese, shredded
- 4 ounces (115 g) Monterey Jack cheese, shredded
- 6 flour tortillas

Directions:

1. In a nonstick skillet, brown beef, onions, and green pepper. Add remaining ingredients except cheese and tortillas to skillet and bring to a boil. Reduce heat. Cover and simmer for 10 minutes. Combine cheeses

in a bowl. In slow cooker, layer about ¾ cup (150 g) beef mixture, 1 tortilla, and about ¼ cup (30 g) cheese. Repeat layers until all ingredients are used. Cover and cook on low 5 to 7 hours.

Nutrition Info:

Per serving: 188 g water; 564 calories (34% from fat, 25% from protein, 41% from carb); 35 g protein; 22 g total fat; 10 g saturated fat; 8 g monounsaturated fat; 1 g polyunsaturated fat; 58 g carb; 14 g fiber; 4 g sugar; 526 mg phosphorus; 341 mg calcium; 7 mg iron; 420 mg sodium; 1241 mg potassium; 490 IU vitamin A; 64 mg ATE vitamin E; 26 mg vitamin C; 67 mg cholesterol

Chili Verde

Servings: 8 Servings

Ingredients:

- 2 tablespoons (28 ml) olive oil
- 1 cup (160 g) diced onion
- 1 teaspoon minced garlic
- 1 pound (455 g) extra-lean ground beef
- ½ pound (225 g) ground pork
- 3 cups (700 ml) low-sodium chicken broth
- 2 cups (475 ml) water
- 8 ounces (225 g) diced green chilies
- 4 large potatoes, diced
- 10 ounces (280 g) frozen corn
- 1 teaspoon black pepper
- ½ teaspoon oregano
- 1 teaspoon cumin

Directions:

1. Heat oil in a skillet over medium-high heat and then brown onion, garlic, beef, and pork. Cook until meat is no longer pink. Combine meat mixture and

remaining ingredients in slow cooker. Cover and cook on low 4 to 6 hours or until potatoes are soft.

Nutrition Info:

Per serving: 422 g water; 414 calories (42% from fat, 20% from protein, 38% from carb); 21 g protein; 20 g total fat; 7 g saturated fat; 9 g monounsaturated fat; 2 g polyunsaturated fat; 40 g carb; 5 g fiber; 4 g sugar; 283 mg phosphorus; 53 mg calcium; 4 mg iron; 234 mg sodium; 1233 mg potassium; 60 IU vitamin A; 1 mg ATE vitamin E; 29 mg vitamin C; 60 mg cholesterol

Meatball Stew

Servings: 8 Servings

Ingredients:

- 2 pounds (900 g) meatballs, basic or turkey
- 6 medium potatoes, cubed
- 1 cup (160 g) sliced onion
- 1½ cups (195 g) sliced carrots
- 1 cup (240 g) low-sodium ketchup
- 1 cup (235 ml) water
- 2 tablespoons (28 ml) vinegar
- 1 teaspoon basil
- 1 teaspoon oregano
- ¼ teaspoon pepper

Directions:

1. Brown meatballs in skillet over medium heat. Drain. Place potatoes, onion, and carrots in slow cooker. Top with meatballs. Combine ketchup, water, vinegar, basil, oregano, and pepper. Pour over meatballs. Cover and cook on high 4 to 5 hours or until vegetables are tender.

Nutrition Info:

Per serving: 381 g water; 485 calories (29% from fat, 20% from protein, 51% from carb); 25 g protein; 16 g total fat; 6 g saturated fat; 7 g monounsaturated fat; 1 g polyunsaturated fat; 63 g carb; 7 g fiber; 13 g sugar; 355 mg phosphorus; 96 mg calcium; 5 mg iron; 122 mg sodium; 1807 mg potassium; 4418 IU vitamin A; 11 mg ATE vitamin E; 31 mg vitamin C; 60 mg cholesterol

Saucy Beef

Servings: 12 Servings

Ingredients:

- 3 pounds (1 1/3 kg) extra-lean ground beef
- 1 cup (160 g) thinly sliced onions
- 10 ounces (280 g) low-sodium cream of mushroom soup
- 4 ounces (115 g) mushrooms, sliced
- 1½ cups (355 ml) beer
- ½ cup (120 g) low-sodium ketchup
- 1 bay leaf ¼ teaspoon black pepper

Directions:

1. Place meat in slow cooker. Combine remaining ingredients. Pour over meat. Cover and cook on low 7 to 9 hours or on high 4 to 6 hours. Remove bay leaf before serving.

Nutrition Info:

Per serving: 146 g water; 307 calories (60% from fat, 30% from protein, 9% from carb); 22 g protein; 20 g total fat; 8 g saturated fat; 9 g monounsaturated fat; 1 g polyunsaturated fat; 7 g carb; 1

g fiber; 4 g sugar; 191 mg phosphorus; 17 mg calcium; 2 mg iron; 169 mg sodium; 506 mg potassium; 96 IU vitamin A; 1 mg ATE vitamin E; 3 mg vitamin C; 79 mg cholesterol

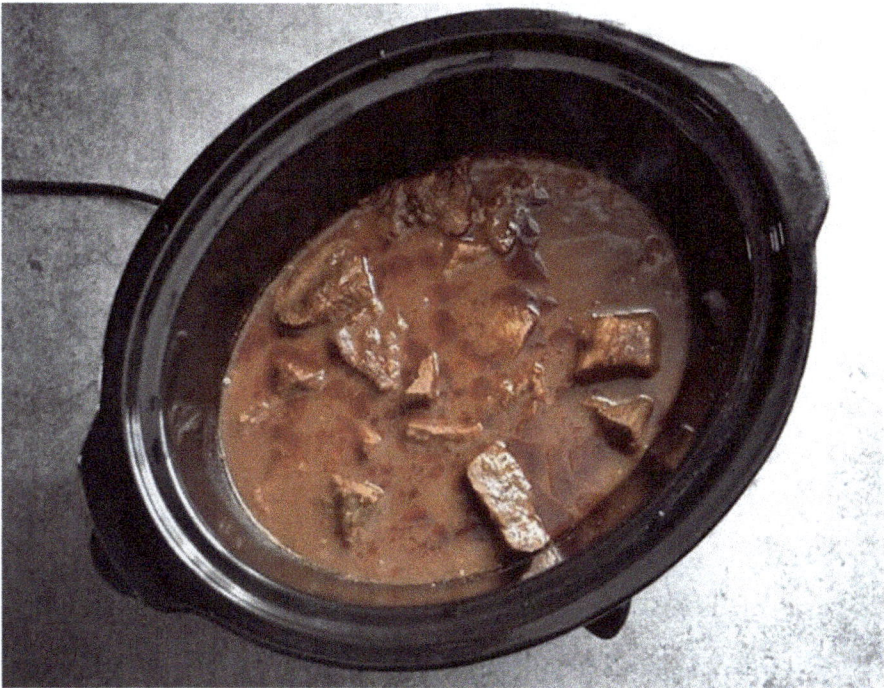

Italian Rice Casserole

Servings: 8 Servings

Ingredients:

- 1 pound (455 g) ground beef
- 1 cup (160 g) chopped onion
- 3 cups (555 g) uncooked long-grain rice
- 3 cups (735 g) no-salt-added tomato sauce
- 1 teaspoon Italian seasoning
- ½ teaspoon minced garlic
- 6 ounces (170 g) mozzarella, shredded
- 1 cup (225 g) low-fat cottage cheese
- 4 cups (950 ml) water

Directions:

1. Place ground beef and chopped onion in a nonstick skillet. Brown over medium-high heat and then drain. Combine beef mixture and remaining ingredients in slow cooker. Cover and cook on high for 6 hours or until the rice is tender.

Nutrition Info:

Per serving: 295 g water; 508 calories (26% from fat, 21% from protein, 53% from carb); 26 g protein; 14 g total fat; 7 g saturated fat; 5 g monounsaturated fat; 1 g polyunsaturated fat; 66 g carb; 3 g fiber; 5 g sugar; 336 mg phosphorus; 232 mg calcium; 5 mg iron; 302 mg sodium; 658 mg potassium; 451 IU vitamin A; 32 mg ATE vitamin E; 14 mg vitamin C; 55 mg cholesterol

Spanish Rice Meal

Servings: 6 Servings

Ingredients:

- 2 pounds (900 g) lean ground beef, browned
- 1 cup (150 g) chopped green bell pepper
- 1 cup (160 g) chopped onion
- 2 teaspoons Worcestershire sauce
- 2 teaspoons chili powder
- 1 can (6 ounces, or 170 g) tomato paste
- 1 can (28 ounces, or 785 g) crushed tomatoes
- 1 cup (185 g) uncooked long-grain rice
- 1 cup (235 ml) water

Directions:

1. Combine all ingredients in slow cooker and cook on low 6 to 8 hours or until rice is done.

Nutrition Info:

Per serving: 331 g water; 537 calories (45% from fat, 25% from protein, 30% from carb); 33 g protein; 27 g total fat; 10 g saturated fat; 11 g monounsaturated fat; 1 g polyunsaturated fat; 41 g carb; 4 g fiber; 5 g sugar; 321 mg phosphorus; 48 mg

calcium; 6 mg iron; 365 mg sodium; 1158 mg potassium; 1598 IU vitamin A; 0 mg ATE vitamin E; 66 mg vitamin C; 104 mg cholesterol

Hamburger Casserole

Servings: 4 Servings

Ingredients:

- 3 potatoes, sliced
- 1 cup (130 g) sliced carrots
- 1 cup (160 g) sliced onion
- ½ teaspoon pepper
- 1 pound (455 g) ground beef, browned and drained
- 2 cups (475 ml) low-sodium tomato juice

Directions:

1. Combine all ingredients in slow cooker. Cover and cook on low 6 to 8 hours.

Nutrition Info:

Per serving: 474 g water; 509 calories (35% from fat, 22% from protein, 43% from carb); 28 g protein; 20 g total fat; 8 g saturated fat; 8 g monounsaturated fat; 1 g polyunsaturated fat; 56 g carb; 7 g fiber; 10 g sugar; 373 mg phosphorus; 68 mg calcium; 5 mg iron; 127 mg sodium; 2021 mg potassium; 5959 IU vitamin A; 0 mg ATE vitamin E; 51 mg vitamin C; 78 mg cholesterol

Pizza Burgers

Servings: 4 Servings

Ingredients:

- 1 pound (455 g) extra-lean ground beef
- ½ cup (80 g) chopped onions
- ¼ teaspoon pepper
- 1 cup (245 g) low-sodium spaghetti sauce
- 1 cup (115 g) shredded mozzarella cheese

Directions:

1. Brown ground beef and onion in a skillet over medium-high heat. Drain. Add remaining ingredients to skillet and mix well. Pour into slow cooker. Cover and cook on low 1 to 2 hours.

Nutrition Info:

Per serving: 146 g water; 419 calories (61% from fat, 28% from protein, 11% from carb); 29 g protein; 28 g total fat; 12 g saturated fat; 12 g monounsaturated fat; 1 g polyunsaturated fat; 12 g carb; 2 g fiber; 8 g sugar; 285 mg phosphorus; 170 mg calcium; 3 mg iron; 268 mg sodium; 591 mg potassium; 544 IU vitamin A; 49 mg ATE vitamin E; 8 mg vitamin C; 100 mg cholesterol

Cincinnati Spaghetti Casserole

Servings: 8 Servings

Ingredients:

- ½ cup (80 g) chopped onions
- 2 cups (475 ml) low-sodium tomato juice
- 2 teaspoons chili powder
- ½ cup (58 g) shredded Cheddar cheese
- 1½ pounds (680 g) extra-lean ground beef, browned
- 12 ounces (340 g) spaghetti, cooked

Directions:

1. Combine all ingredients in slow cooker. Cover and cook on low 4 hours. Check mixture about halfway through the cooking time. If it's becoming dry, stir in an additional 1 cup (235 ml) of tomato juice.

Nutrition Info:

Per serving: 151 g water; 301 calories (52% from fat, 28% from protein, 20% from carb); 21 g protein; 18 g total fat; 8 g saturated fat; 7 g monounsaturated fat; 1 g polyunsaturated fat; 15 g carb; 3 g fiber; 3 g sugar; 216 mg phosphorus; 82 mg calcium; 3 mg iron; 121 mg sodium; 434 mg potassium; 543 IU

vitamin A; 21 mg ATE vitamin E; 12 mg vitamin C; 67 mg
cholesterol

Rice With Beef And Peppers

Servings: 6 Servings

Ingredients:

- 1 pound (455 g) ground beef
- 1 cup (150 g) coarsely chopped green bell pepper
- 1 cup (150 g) coarsely chopped red bell pepper
- 1 cup (160 g) chopped onion
- 1 cup (190 g) brown rice
- 3 cups (700 ml) low-sodium beef broth
- 1 tablespoon (15 ml) reduced-sodium soy sauce

Directions:

1. Brown beef in skillet over medium-high heat. Drain. Combine beef and remaining ingredients in slow cooker and mix well. Cover and cook on low 5 to 6 hours or on high 3 hours until liquid is absorbed.

Nutrition Info:

Per serving: 260 g water; 245 calories (50% from fat, 28% from protein, 21% from carb); 17 g protein; 14 g total fat; 5 g saturated fat; 6 g monounsaturated fat; 1 g polyunsaturated fat; 13 g carb; 2 g fiber; 3 g sugar; 171 mg phosphorus; 27 mg calcium; 2 mg

iron; 133 mg sodium; 433 mg potassium; 870 IU vitamin A; 0 mg ATE vitamin E; 54 mg vitamin C; 52 mg cholesterol

Taco Bake

Servings: 6 Servings

Ingredients:

- 1½ pounds (680 g) extra-lean ground beef, browned
- 1 can (14 ounces, or 400 g) no-salt-added diced tomatoes
- 4 ounces (115 g) diced green chilies
- 2 tablespoons (15 g) Salt-Free Mexican Seasoning
- ¼ cup (60 ml) water
- 6 corn tortillas, cut in ½-inch (1.3 cm) strips
- ½ cup (115 g) fat-free sour cream
- 1 cup (115 g) shredded Cheddar cheese

Directions:

1. Combine beef, tomatoes, chilies, Mexican seasoning, and water in slow cooker. Stir in tortilla strips. Cover and cook on low 7 to 8 hours. Spread sour cream over casserole. Sprinkle with cheese. Cover and let stand 5 minutes until cheese melts.

Nutrition Info:

Per serving: 194 g water; 437 calories (61% from fat, 27% from protein, 12% from carb); 29 g protein; 30 g total fat; 14 g saturated fat; 11 g monounsaturated fat; 1 g polyunsaturated fat; 13 g carb; 2 g fiber; 2 g sugar; 365 mg phosphorus; 230 mg calcium; 3 mg iron; 312 mg sodium; 550 mg potassium; 397 IU vitamin A; 77 mg ATE vitamin E; 13 mg vitamin C; 109 mg cholesterol

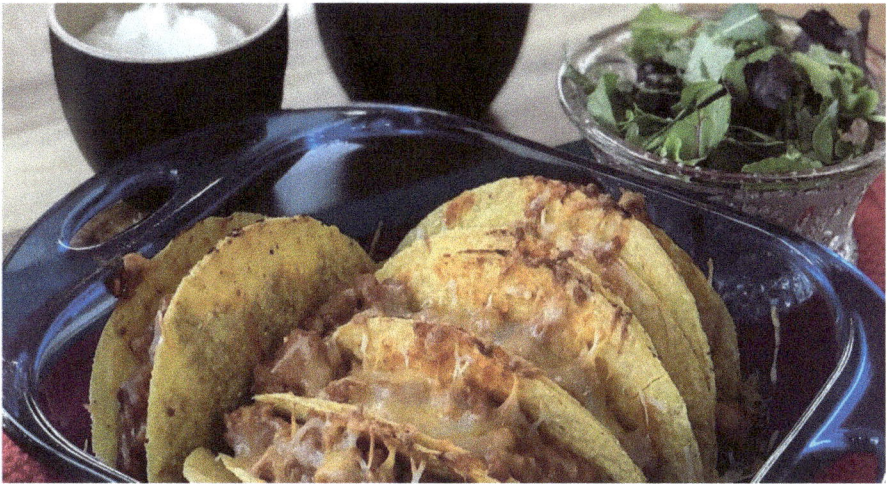

Beef And Cabbage Casserole

Servings: 4 Servings

Ingredients:

- 1 tablespoon (15 ml) olive oil
- 1 cup (160 g) chopped onion
- 1 pound (455 g) extra-lean ground beef
- ¼ teaspoon pepper
- 3 cups (210 g) shredded cabbage
- 1 can (10 ounces, or 280 g) reduced-sodium condensed tomato soup

Directions:

1. Heat oil in a skillet over medium-high heat. Sauté onion and then add ground beef and brown. Season with pepper. Layer half of cabbage in slow cooker, followed by half of meat mixture. Repeat layers. Pour soup over top. Cover and cook on low 3 to 4 hours.

Nutrition Info:

Per serving: 233 g water; 353 calories (60% from fat, 26% from protein, 14% from carb); 23 g protein; 23 g total fat; 8 g saturated fat; 11 g monounsaturated fat; 1 g polyunsaturated fat;

12 g carb; 2 g fiber; 6 g sugar; 199 mg phosphorus; 47 mg calcium; 3 mg iron; 103 mg sodium; 571 mg potassium; 259 IU vitamin A; 4 mg ATE vitamin E; 47 mg vitamin C; 78 mg cholesterol

Meaty Spaghetti Sauce

Servings: 8 Servings

Ingredients:

- 1 pound (455 g) lean ground beef
- ½ pound (225 g) Italian sausage
- 1 can (28 ounces, or 785 g) no-salt-added diced tomatoes, undrained
- 1 can (6 ounces, or 170 g) no-salt-added tomato paste
- 8 ounces (225 g) mushrooms, sliced
- 1 cup (160 g) chopped onion
- ¾ cup (113 g) chopped green bell pepper
- ½ cup (120 ml) dry red wine
- 1/3 cup (80 ml) water
- 2¼ ounces (64 g) ripe olives, drained and sliced
- 2 teaspoons sugar
- ½ teaspoon Worcestershire sauce
- ½ teaspoon chili powder
- ¼ teaspoon black pepper
- ½ teaspoon minced garlic

Directions:

1. In a large skillet, cook ground beef and sausage over medium heat until brown. Drain off fat. Transfer meat mixture to a slow cooker. Stir in remaining ingredients. Cover and cook on low for 9 to 10 hours or on high for 4½ to 5 hours.

Nutrition Info:

Per serving: 246 g water; 309 calories (59% from fat, 23% from protein, 18% from carb); 18 g protein; 20 g total fat; 7 g saturated fat; 9 g monounsaturated fat; 2 g polyunsaturated fat; 14 g carb; 3 g fiber; 8 g sugar; 194 mg phosphorus; 64 mg calcium; 4 mg iron; 164 mg sodium; 805 mg potassium; 571 IU vitamin A; 0 mg ATE vitamin E; 29 mg vitamin C; 61 mg cholesterol

Pork Chops In Beer

Servings: 6 Servings

Ingredients:

- 1 tablespoon (15 ml) olive oil
- 6 pork loin chops
- 2 cups (320 g) chopped onion
- 12 ounces (355 ml) beer
- 1 teaspoon thyme

Directions:

1. Heat oil in a large skillet over medium-high heat and brown chops on both sides. Place onions in slow cooker and then place chops over top. Combine beer and thyme and pour over chops. Cover and cook on low for 8 to 10 hours or on high for 4 to 5 hours.

Nutrition Info:

Per serving: 174 g water; 195 calories (34% from fat, 50% from protein, 16% from carb); 22 g protein; 7 g total fat; 2 g saturated fat; 4 g monounsaturated fat; 1 g polyunsaturated fat; 7 g carb; 1 g fiber; 2 g sugar; 244 mg phosphorus; 31 mg calcium; 1 mg

iron; 56 mg sodium; 468 mg potassium; 14 IU vitamin A; 2 mg ATE vitamin E; 5 mg vitamin C; 64 mg cholesterol

Creamy Beef Burgundy

Servings: 8 Servings

Ingredients:

- 4 pounds (1.8 g) beef round roast
- 1 can (10 ounces, or 280 g) low-sodium cream of mushroom soup
- 1 cup (235 ml) burgundy wine
- 1 cup (160 g) finely chopped onion
- 1 tablespoon (1.3 g) dried parsley

Directions:

1. Place meat in slow cooker. Blend soup and wine together in a mixing bowl. Pour over meat. Top with onion and parsley. Cover and cook on low 5 hours or until meat is tender but not dry. Serve the sauce as gravy over the sliced or cubed meat.

Nutrition Info:

Per serving: 241 g water; 342 calories (26% from fat, 67% from protein, 7% from carb); 51 g protein; 9 g total fat; 3 g saturated fat; 4 g monounsaturated fat; 1 g polyunsaturated fat; 6 g carb; 1 g fiber; 2 g sugar; 523 mg phosphorus; 60 mg calcium; 5 mg

iron; 279 mg sodium; 1020 mg potassium; 43 IU vitamin A; 1 mg ATE vitamin E; 2 mg vitamin C; 114 mg cholesterol

4-WEEK MEAL PLAN

Week 1

Monday
Breakfast: Tofu Frittata
Lunch: Pork Chops In Beer
Dinner: Stewed Tomatoes

Tuesday
Breakfast: Tapioca
Lunch: Creamy Beef Burgundy
Dinner: Oregano Salad

Wednesday
Breakfast: Fruit Oats
Lunch: Smothered Steak
Dinner: Black Beans With Corn Kernels

Thursday
Breakfast: Grapefruit Mix
Lunch: Pork For Sandwiches
Dinner: Stuffed Acorn Squash

Friday
Breakfast: Berry Yogurt
Lunch: Cranberry Pork Roast

Dinner: Greek Eggplant

Saturday
Breakfast: Soft Pudding
Lunch: Pan-asian Pot Roast
Dinner: Thyme Sweet Potatoes

Sunday
Breakfast: Black Beans Salad
Lunch: Short Ribs
Dinner: Barley Vegetable Soup

Week 2

Monday
Breakfast: Carrot Pudding
Lunch: French Dip
Dinner: Butter Corn

Tuesday
Breakfast: Apple Cake
Lunch: Italian Roast With Vegetables
Dinner: Orange Glazed Carrots

Wednesday
Breakfast: Almond Milk Barley Cereals
Lunch: Honey Mustard Ribs
Dinner: Cinnamon Acorn Squash

Thursday

Breakfast: Cashews Cake

Lunch: Pizza Casserole

Dinner: Glazed Root Vegetables

Friday

Breakfast: Artichoke Frittata

Lunch: Hawaiian Pork Roast

Dinner: Stir Fried Steak, Shiitake And Asparagus

Saturday

Breakfast: Mexican Eggs

Lunch: Apple Cranberry Pork Roast

Dinner: Cilantro Brussel Sprouts

Sunday

Breakfast: Stewed Peach

Lunch: Swiss Steak

Dinner: Italian Zucchini

Week 3

Monday

Breakfast: Lamb Cassoule t

Lunch: Glazed Pork Roast

Dinner: Cilantro Parsnip Chunks

Tuesday

Breakfast: Fruited Tapioca

Lunch: Swiss Steak In Wine Sauce

Dinner: Corn Casserole

Wednesday

Breakfast: Baby Spinach Shrimp Salad

Lunch: Italian Pork Chops

Dinner: Pilaf With Bella Mushrooms

Thursday

Breakfast: Coconut And Fruit Cake

Lunch: Italian Pot Roast

Dinner: Italian Style Yellow Squash

Friday

Breakfast: Apple And Squash Bowls

Lunch: Beef With Horseradish Sauce

Dinner: Stevia Peas With Marjoram

Saturday

Breakfast: Slow Cooker Chocolate Cake

Lunch: Oriental Pot Roast

Dinner: Broccoli Rice Casserole

Sunday

Breakfast: Fish Omelet

Lunch: Barbecued Ribs

Dinner: Italians Style Mushroom Mix

Week 4

Monday
Breakfast: Brown Cake
Lunch: Ham And Scalloped Pota toes
Dinner: Broccoli Casserole

Tuesday
Breakfast: Stevia And Walnuts Cut Oats
Lunch: Pork And Pineapple Roast

Wednesday
Breakfast: Walnut And Cinnamon Oatmeal
Lunch: Barbecued Brisket
Dinner: Dinner: Slow Cooker Lasagna

Thursday
Breakfast: Tender Rosemary Sweet Potatoes
Lunch: Barbecued Short Ribs
Dinner: Brussels Sprouts Casserole

Friday
Breakfast: Orange And Maple Syrup Quinoa
Lunch: Beer-braised Short Ribs
Dinner: Pasta And Mushrooms

Saturday
Breakfast: Vanilla And Nutmeg Oatmeal
Lunch: Lamb Stew
Dinner: Onion Cabbage

Sunday

Breakfast: Pecans Cake

Lunch: Barbecued Ham

Dinner: Cheese Broccoli

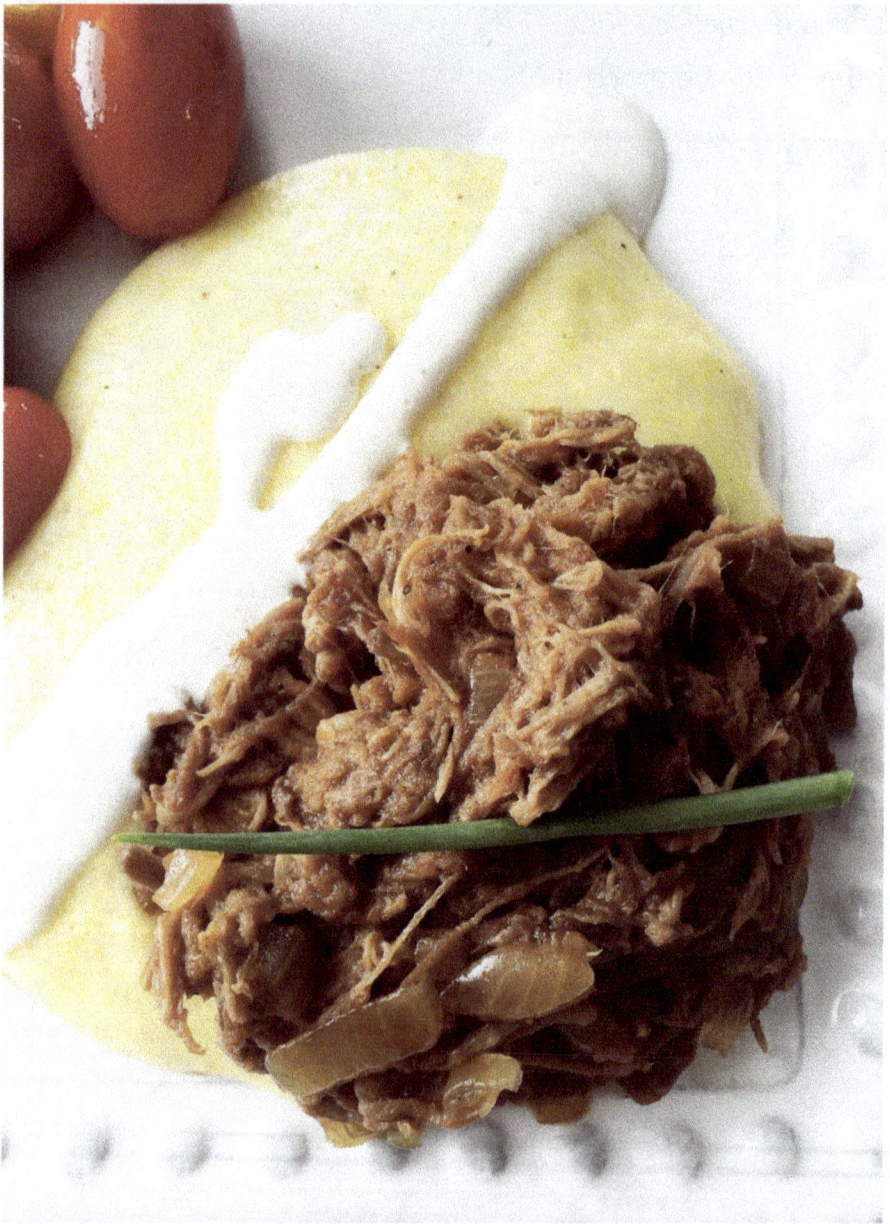

www.ingramcontent.com/pod-product-compliance
Lightning Source LLC
Chambersburg PA
CBHW050755030426
42336CB00012B/1837